LIFE QUOTES

My Counseling Success and Perspective as a Client with Bipolar

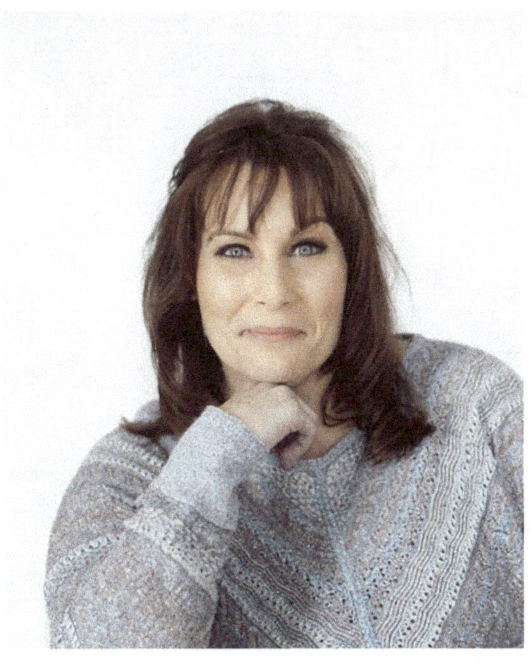

Jodie Hansohn

LIFE QUOTES

My Counseling Success and Perspective as a Client with Bipolar

Jodie Hansohn

A BOOK OF QUOTES FOR CLIENTS

A GUIDE OF QUOTES TO USE EVERYDAY
TO HELP YOU WITH EFFECTIVE COUNSELING

A BOOK OF QUOTES FOR CLIENTS

www.instagram.com/noexcusbipolar

DEDICATION

This book is dedicated to Mrs. Annetta Benjamin, Owner of Benjamin Counseling Center, LLC.
The most extraordinary counselor one could ever have the opportunity to work with. Thank you for always believing in me and for never giving up on me! Thanks for always setting me straight! Through our 13 years of successful counseling, you have given me the tools, and
techniques that were used to help guide me and teach me how to live a successful life. I would not be who I am as a client, as a wife, as a mother, as a sibling or as a friend had it not been for your help. As I learned to successfully navigate my illness through counseling and by using my tools and techniques. Therefore, I decided that I would put together a book of quotes that are everyday helpers that I learned to work with by journaling them and putting them into practice for everyday guidance. In doing so these were the words that not only I realized were being used by me but were being taught through all my counseling sessions throughout the years. I also learned to use them in my daily journaling. This has led me to an incredibly happy, healthy, and successful life. This book is also being dedicated to every client and staff member at Benjamin Counseling Center, MA, LPC, NCC.

Table of Contents

IMPORTANT MESSAGE

(How to Read This Book of Counselor and Client Quotes)

As you read each quote, you will start to notice and remember, that these are all the words used and exercised with you in your counseling sessions. You will begin to see that when you say them, practice them, and journal them, that they are all your actions, feelings, thoughts, helpers, and hurts. At the end of each quote, I have also included a personal example of how each quote should be used.

As I am being honest with you, I hope that the each of you, will learn to perfect these words and meanings, in hopes that they will become the key to your success.

MY MOTTO "NO EXCUSES"

"There are absolutely no excuses to have excuses!"
Jodie Hansohn

As I learned to perfect my illness through counseling and using my tools and techniques, I decided that I would put together a book of quotes that are everyday helpers! Through counseling I learned to journal and put into action how life should be lived. Now I am looking to help others better themselves and to strive for nothing but the best. In doing so, these were the words that not only I realized were being used by me but were also being taught through all my counseling sessions. Throughout the years I learned to perfect them, and it has led me to a happy place that I call life.

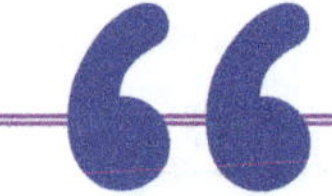

ACCEPTANCE
(Reality & The Truth)

"In human psychology is a person's assent to the reality of a situation, recognizing a process or condition often a negative or uncomfortable situation, without attempting to change it or protest it."

Wikipedia

My Perspective

I have accepted and conquered the Bipolar Illness.

Jodie Hansohn

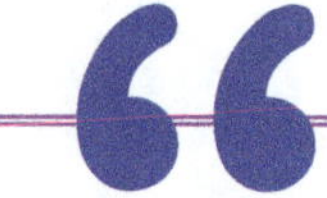

ACCOUNTABILITY
(Always be accountable)

"No individual can achieve worthy goals without accepting accountability for his or her own actions."

Dan Miller

My Perspective

I take accountability for being at the wrong place when my rape happened.

Jodie Hansohn

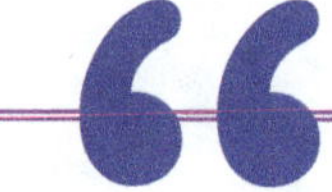

ACTIONS

(For every action there is a reaction, good or bad)

"Life isn't always about doing the things we like to do. It's about doing things we have to do."

David Goggins

My Perspective

My actions choose my outcomes.

Jodie Hansohn

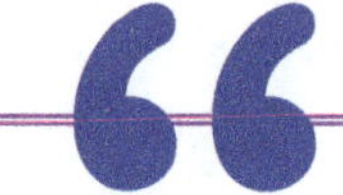

APPOINTMENTS
(Keep your appointments)

"Unfaithfulness in the keeping of an appointment is an act of clear dishonesty. You may as well borrow a person's money as his time. A wise woman never yields by appointment."

Greg Abbott

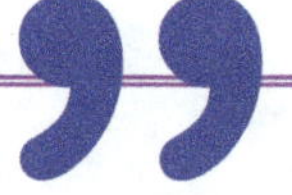

My Perspective

I do not miss my counseling appointments.

Jodie Hansohn

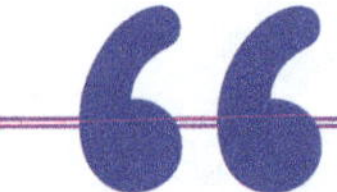

THE BUDDY SYSTEM
(Use your buddy system)

"Networking is a lot like nutrition and fitness: we know what to do, the hard part is making it a top priority."

Herminia Ibarra

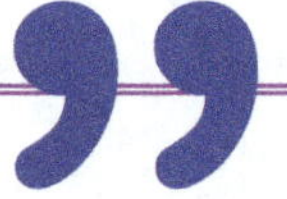

My Perspective

I use my journaling to clear my head.
I stay in touch with my doctors to keep informed. I never miss a day of my medication. I do not drink or do drugs. I choose to stay happy and healthy.

Jodie Hansohn

COUNSELING
(Always counsel)

"Not seeking counseling when you know you need it is in fact a sign of weakness and timidity."

Samuel Zulu

"It is not fair to ask of others, what you or not willing to do yourself"

Eleanor Roosevelt

My Perspective

I counsel because my illness requires the cognitive therapy. (I stay accountable to myself so I can hold others accountable as well.)

Jodie Hansohn

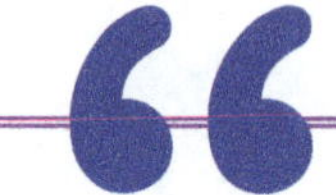

CHOICES

(Choose wisely)

"Life is a matter of choices, and every choice you make makes you"

John Maxwell

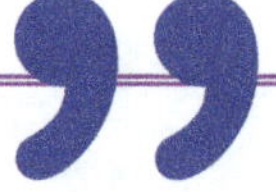

My Perspective

I chose to continue to educate myself about my illness, and to make the healthy choices that are required to take care of my illness.

Jodie Hansohn

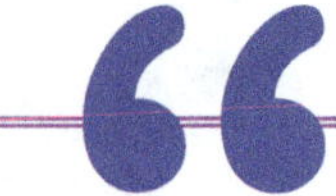

COGNITIVE THERAPY
(Overcoming difficulties and meeting your goals)

"Happiness is not dependent on the good or bad opinions of others, but instead upon your actions."

Lawrence Wallace

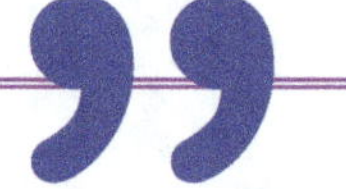

(The Principle of cognitive behavioral therapy)

The first principle of cognitive therapy is that the majority of your moods are created by your thoughts, perceptions, attitudes, and beliefs about a situation. They are not caused by the actual situation itself.

My Perspective

I choose cognitive therapy because it is one of the keys to the treatment and success of my illness.

Jodie Hansohn

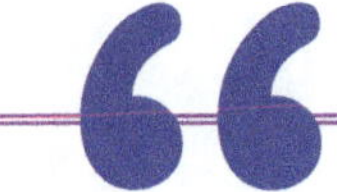

CONSISTENCY
(Practice accuracy)

"Success isn't always about greatness. It's about consistency." "Consistent hard challenging work leads to success. Greatness will come."

Dwayne Johnson

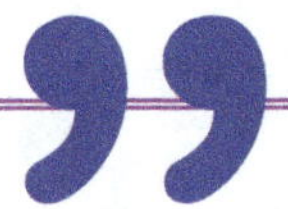

My Perspective

I am consistent every day with the same routine, of taking my medications, exercising, and dieting.

Jodie Hansohn

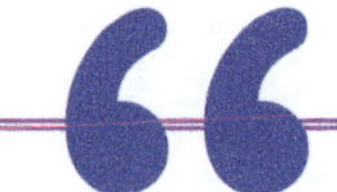

CONTROL
(Control your daily life)

"You only have control over three things in your life- the thoughts you think, the images you visualize, and the actions you take"

Jack Canfield

My Perspective

I control my actions by journaling. Instead reacting I choose to respond.

Jodie Hansohn

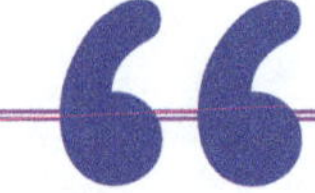

CRAZY
(Words and Actions)

I believe that if you act crazy you are crazy.

Jodie Hansohn

My Perspective

If I scream and act out, then I am acting crazy. Learn to use your words appropriately.

Jodie Hansohn

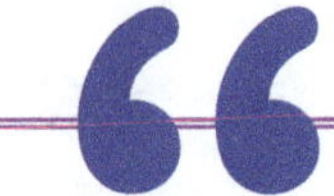

EXERCISE

(Feeling good)

"True enjoyment comes from activity of the mind and exercise of the body; the two are forever united."

Thomas Jefferson

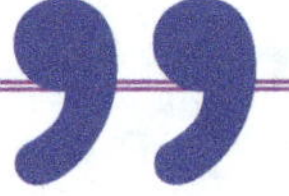

My Perspective

I always go for a run or a walk. (It creates my peace of mind.)

Jodie Hansohn

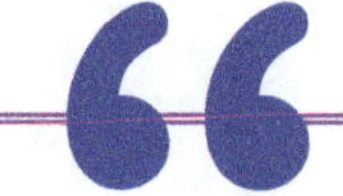

EXCUSES
(There are "No Excuses")

"Excuses are the lies you convince yourself are true to avoid proving you are worthy of the gift you were given. Say this with me, no more excuses."

Steve Harvey

My Perspective

I do not make excuses. I live by facts and truth.

Jodie Hansohn

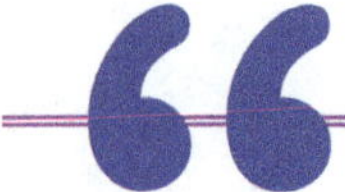

FEELINGS/EMOTIONS

(Be in tune with your feelings and emotions)

"If you take control of your behavior, your emotions will fall into place."

"When you control your thoughts and emotions, you control everything."

John C. Maxwell

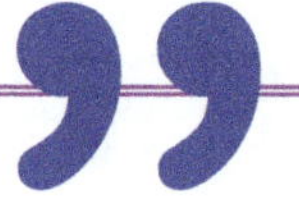

My Perspective

I keep my emotions and feelings in check. I counsel, journal, and continue with my cognitive therapy.

Jodie Hansohn

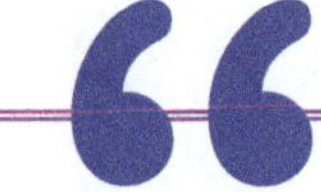

HURTS

(Know your hurts)

"The pain of yesterday is the strength of today."

Paulo Coelho

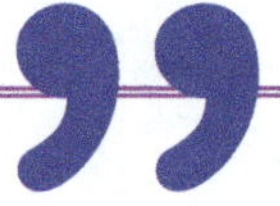

My Perspective

I allow myself to feel the hurt. I do not run or hide, instead I counsel to learn and grow.

Jodie Hansohn

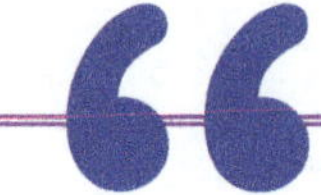

HELPERS

(Your plan of action)

"In life we have Helpers and Hurts, choose to Help yourself every day."

Annetta Benjamin, LPC

My Perspective

I will call and make extra counseling appointments,
I will not participate in bad behaviors.

Jodie Hansohn

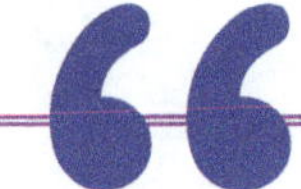

HEALTH
(You are in charge of your health)

"Is an investment not an expense"

Freshly

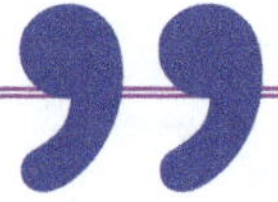

My Perspective

I take accountability for how I look, by the way I eat, exercise, and take care of my illness.

Jodie Hansohn

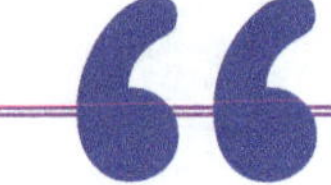

HONESTY
(Stop lying)

"The high road is always respected. Honesty and integrity are always rewarded."

Scott Hamilton

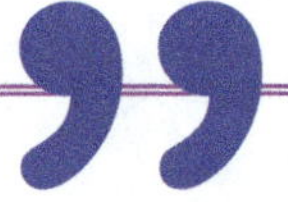

My Perspective

I started with honesty, because I wanted to know what was wrong with me and how could I change and become the best of me.

Jodie Hansohn

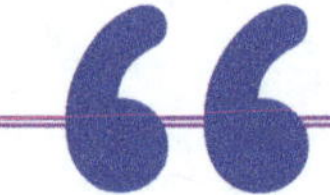

ILLNESS

(A disease or period of sickness affecting the body or mind)

"The strongest people I've met have not been given an easier life. They've learned to create strength and happiness from dark places."

Kristen Butler

My Perspective

I took it upon myself to find out what in the hell was wrong with me and I own it.

Jodie Hansohn

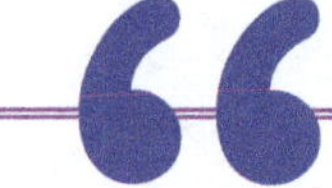

THE ONION

(Peel the onion)

"Acting is like peeling an onion. You have to peel away each layer to reveal another."

Juliette Binoche

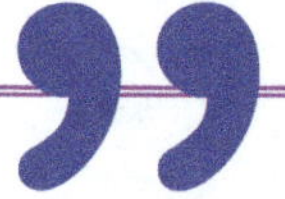

My Perspective

Through cognitive counseling, I have learned to peel the layers of hurt, and truths, for an effective goal in life to be safe, healthy, and happy with a lifetime of success.

Jodie Hansohn

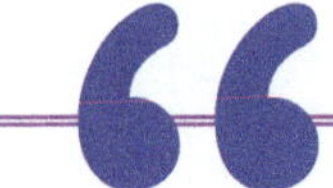

SAFE PLACE
(Know your safe place)

"The ache for home lives in all of us, it is the safe place where we can go as we are and not be questioned."

Maya Angelou

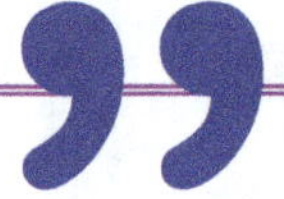

My Perspective

I go to my bedroom for my safe place.

Jodie Hansohn

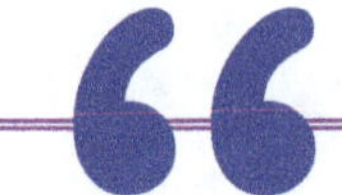

JOURNAL

(Journal your feelings, thoughts, behavior, helpers, and hurts)

"I can recapture everything when I write my thoughts, my ideas and my fantasies."

Natalie Goldberg

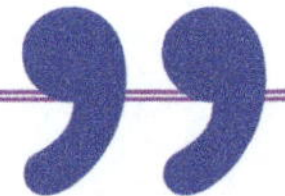

My Perspective

I journal. I journal all my hurt, hate, and anger. It might be filthy, but it is all out of my head.

Jodie Hansohn

LIFE

(You are in control of your life)

"You are the only person who thinks in your mind! You are the power and authority in your world."

Louise L. Hay

My Perspective

I control my life by the way I think and the choices I make.

Jodie Hansohn

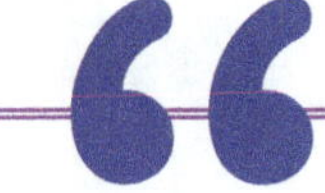

NUTRITION
(Food)

"The food you eat can be either the safest and most powerful form of medicine or the slowest form of poison."

Ann Wigmore

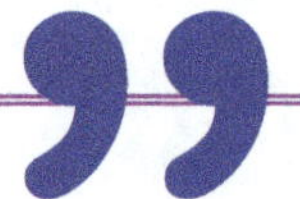

My Perspective

I choose to find a doctor who specialized in bipolar, metabolic syndrome, and I have learned that the many different things that I eat, will affect my illness.

Jodie Hansohn

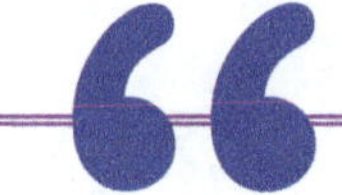

PREPARE

(Prepare to do your absolute best)

"The best preparation for tomorrow, is doing your best today."

Premier protein

My Perspective

I prepare everyday by journaling throughout the day the good, the bad, and the ugly.

Jodie Hansohn

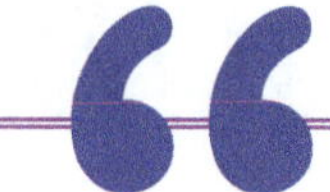

SELF CARE
(Improve your health and well-being)

"The body can endure practically anything – pain, fatigue, you name it – but it's the mind that matters."

Dave Pelzer

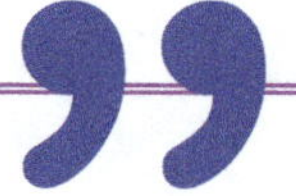

My Perspective

Self care is taking accountability. I come first before anyone.

Jodie Hansohn

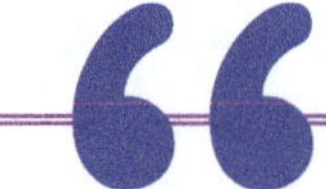

SUCCESS

(You are in charge of your success)

"Success is the sum of small efforts repeated day in and day out."

Robert Collier

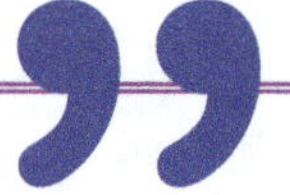

My Perspective

I am the success of my illness, by learning to master it.

Jodie Hansohn

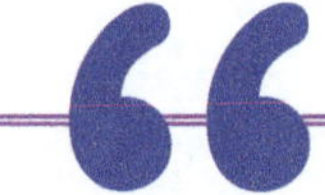

SPIRAL
(Spiraling out of control)

"There are those that handle mental illness with responsibility while others spiral out of control"

Steven Magee

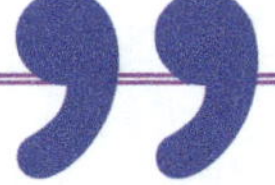

My Perspective

Spiraling out of control holds no accountability. I go to my safe place and journal, or I take my anger and put it into a workout. Do not Spiral out of control.

Jodie Hansohn

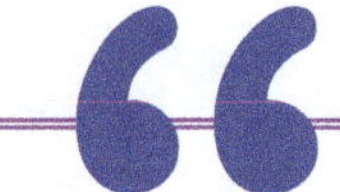

TRIGGERS
(Know your triggers)

"Triggers are like little psychic explosions that crash through avoidance and bring the dissociated, avoided trauma suddenly, unexpectedly, back into consciousness."

Carolyn Spring

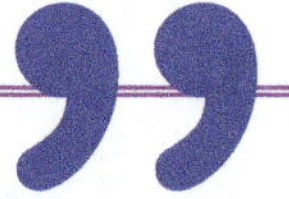

My Perspective

I know who I can spend quality time with and who I absolutely cannot.

Jodie Hansohn

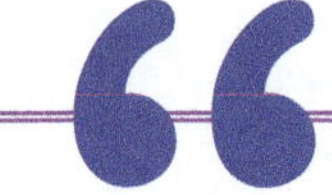

TEMPORARY
(Not permanent)

*"Everything passes. Joy. Pain. The moment of triumph; the sigh of despair.
Nothing lasts forever -not even this."*

Paul Stewart

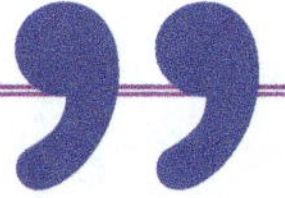

My Perspective

I have spent 13 years in counseling to perfect my illness and to forgive myself for the mistakes that I have made.
I learned to forgive the person who raped me.

Jodie Hansohn

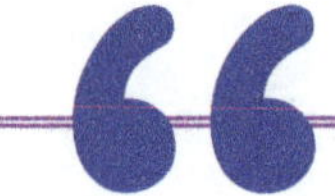

THOUGHTS
(Action or Process)

"Clear thinking requires courage rather than intelligence."

Thomas Szasz

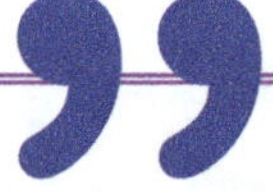

My Perspective

I choose to think positively, and journal the hurt and anger. I have learned what triggers me.

Jodie Hansohn

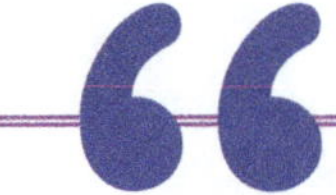

TIME MANAGEMENT

(The process of planning and exercising control)

"Gain control of your time, and you will gain control of your life."

John Landis Mason

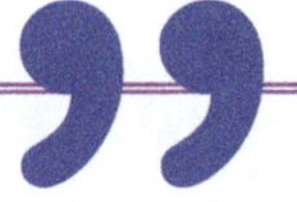

My Perspective

I use time management with everything I do. Eat, exercise, counsel, doctors, journal, and medications. Make it your daily routine.

Jodie Hansohn

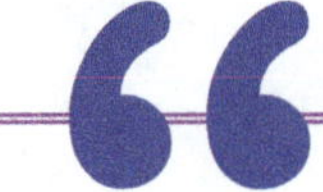

WORDS
(Mean things)

"Sticks and stones may break my bones, but words will always hurt me."

Stephen Fry

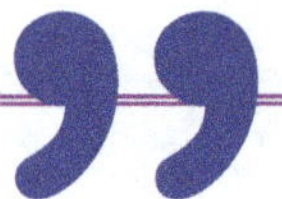

My Perspective

I choose my words carefully; I cannot take back the hurtful things I say.

Jodie Hansohn

MY MOTTO "NO EXCUSES"

There are absolutely no excuses to have excuses!

Jodie Hansohn

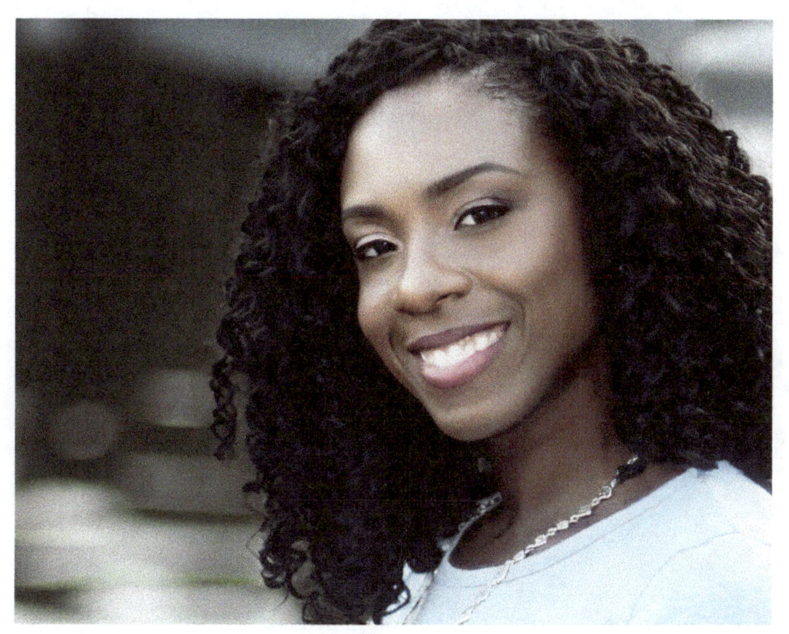

Please remember:
I could not have done this without Mrs. Annetta Benjamin, LPC

Don't forget to check out the book:
5 HELPERS 5 HURTS
A Guide To Improve Your Thoughts and Feelings

www.ingramcontent.com/pod-product-compliance
Lightning Source LLC
LaVergne TN
LVHW050424160826
845677LV00002BA/529

* 9 7 9 8 8 4 6 1 6 1 3 9 9 *